# The Ultimate Air Fry Cookbook for Diabeti

*Easy and Crispy Recipes*
*To Live Well and Control Diabete*

Lilith Ballard

## Table of Contents

# *CAJUN SAUSAGE*

**Preparation Time:** 5 minutes

**Cooking Time:** 20-25 minutes

**Servings:** 4

## Nutritional values:

- Calories: 126 kcal
- Fat: 4.4 g
- Carbohydrates: 11.3 g
- Proteins: 11.2 g

## Ingredients:

- 2 tsp. fresh leaves only or ½ tsp. dried thyme
- 2 tsp. Tabasco sauce
- Chopped sage (optional)
- 3 tsp. minced garlic
- 2 tsp. maple syrup
- ¼ tsp. sea salt
- ½ tsp. each paprika and cayenne

- 1.5 lbs. ground sausage (chicken sausage or lean pork)
- 1 tsp. onion powder
- 1 tsp. chili flakes
- Herbs to garnish optional

## Directions:

1. Put the ground sausage in a big bowl. It should be chilled. If not, you need to get it chilled before you begin cooking this recipe.
2. You may add additional spices if you feel like it. If you do, it is necessary to mix them evenly.
3. You can now add the Tabasco sauce.
4. Mold them into balls, bearing in mind that they'll shrink when they are cooked.
5. Place the patties on a baking tray that has been lined with parchment paper to prevent sticking.
6. If you want them to be crispy, you have to air fry them in batches. Place 5 patties in your air fryer basket at a time.
7. Air fry the patties at 370°F for about 20 minutes. After 10 minutes of cooking, pull out the tray to turn the patties over.
8. After about 20 minutes, the sausage should be ready for consumption. Remove it and air fry the next batch of patties.
9. Serve the sausage with some Tabasco sauce or any other sauce that you prefer.

# *FISH AND CHIPS*

**Preparation Time:** 15 minutes

**Cooking Time:** 31 minutes

**Servings:** 4

## Nutritional values:

- Calories: 415 kcal
- Fat: 7 g
- Carbohydrates: 46 g
- Proteins: 44 g

## Ingredients:

- Cooking spray
- 4 skinless tilapia fillets
- 2 tbsp. water
- 2 russet potatoes, scrubbed
- 2 large eggs
- ½ cup malt vinegar
- 1 cup whole-wheat panko (Japanese-style breadcrumbs)
- 1 cup all-purpose flour
- 1 ¼ tsp. kosher salt, divided

## Directions:

1.  You need to cut the potatoes into spirals and cook them in batches for them to come out very crispy. So, place the first batch in your air fryer basket. Spray them with cooking spray. Toss them for even coating.

2.  Cook the potatoes for 10 minutes at 375°F. Don't forget to turn them over after 5 minutes. After 10 minutes, they should be crispy and golden brown in color. Remove them and put them in an airtight container to keep them warm. Then you can cook the next batch.

3.  When you have been able to cook them all, you can sprinkle ¼ tsp. of salt on them.

4.  Mix ½ tsp. of salt with flour and stir them together.

5.  Whisk the eggs together with some water in another bowl. Also, mix the remaining salt with panko in the third bowl.

6.  Cut each of the fish fillets into 2 long strips and toss them in the flour mixture. After that, you can now dip the coated fillets in the egg mixture. Finally, dredge them in the panko mixture. Try to spray both sides of each fish fillet with cooking spray.

7.  Now, it is time to cook the fish too. Place them on a single layer in your air fryer basket. Cook them at 375°F for 10 minutes.

8.  When they are done, you can serve the fish along with the potato spirals and 2 tbsp. of malt vinegar.

# AIR-FRYER CAULIFLOWER GNOCCHI WITH MARINARA DIPPING SAUCE

**Preparation Time:** 12 minutes

**Cooking Time:** 8 minutes

**Servings:** 8

## Nutritional values:

- Calories: 159 kcal
- Fat: 9.3 g
- Carbohydrates: 14.1 g
- Proteins: 3 g

## Ingredients:

- 3 tbsp. extra-virgin olive oil, divided
- 2 tbsp. chopped fresh flat-leaf parsley
- 2 packs frozen cauliflower gnocchi
- 1 cup reduced-sodium marinara sauce
- ½ cup grated Parmesan cheese

## Directions:

1. Start the process by preheating your air fryer to 375°F. Mix 1 pack of gnocchi with 1 ½ tbsp. of oil and 2 tbsp. of parmesan together evenly.

2. Spray your air fryer basket with cooking spray before you place the gnocchi mixture in it.

3. Cook it for 3 minutes and turn it over before you cook for another 2 minutes.

4. Repeat the process with the second pack of gnocchi.

5. When it is done, you should sprinkle parsley and the remaining ¼ cup of Parmesan on the gnocchi.

6. It is best served with marinara.

# TURKEY BREAST

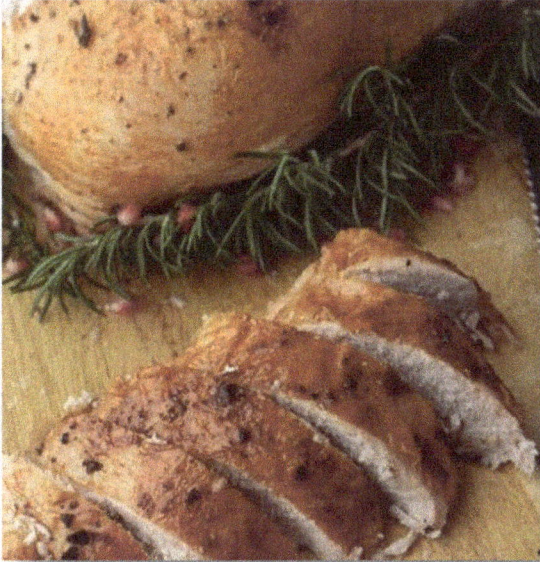

**Preparation Time:** 5 minutes

**Cooking Time:** 55 minutes

**Servings:** 4

**Nutritional values:**

- Calories: 226 kcal
- Fat: 10 g
- Carbohydrates: 2.5 g
- Proteins: 32.5 g

## Ingredients:

- 4 pound turkey breast, with the rib removed
- 2 tsp. kosher salt
- ½ tbsp. dry turkey or poultry seasoning
- 1 tbsp. olive oil

## Directions:

1. Coat the turkey breast with ½ tbsp. of oil.
2. The next step is to season both sides of the turkey breast with salt and turkey seasoning. You can add the remaining oil to the seasoned turkey.
3. Preheat your air fryer to 350°F before cooking the turkey for 20 minutes.
4. Turn it over and cook it at 160°C for another 30 to 35 minutes.
5. Let it cool for 10 minutes before you carve it.

# *POPCORN SHRIMP*

**Preparation Time:** 9 minutes

**Cooking Time:** 22 minutes

**Servings:** 4

## Nutritional values:

- Calories: 297 kcal
- Fat: 3.8 g
- Carbohydrates: 35.4 g
- Proteins: 29.2 g

## Ingredients:

- Cooking spray
- ½ cup all-purpose flour
- 2 eggs
- 2 tbsp. water
- 1 ½ cups panko breadcrumbs
- 1 tbsp. ground cumin
- 1 tbsp. garlic powder
- 1 pound small shrimp, peeled and deveined

- ½ cup no-salt-added ketchup
- 2 tbsp. chopped chipotle chili in adobo
- 2 tbsp. chopped fresh cilantro
- 2 tbsp. lime juice
- 1/8 tsp. kosher salt

**Directions:**

1. Beat the eggs lightly in a small bowl. After that, you should coat your air fryer basket with cooking spray.
2. Pour the flour in another bowl. Add water to the beaten eggs. Find the third bowl and mix garlic powder, cumin, and panko in it.
3. Position half of the shrimp in your air fryer basket and coat it with your cooking spray.
4. Cook it at 360°F for about 4 minutes. Turn it over and continue to cook it for another 4 minutes. Do the same to the second half of the shrimp.
5. Add salt, lime juice, cilantro, chipotles, and ketchup together in the fourth bowl. This will be the dipping sauce for the shrimp. So, you have to serve the popcorn shrimp with the sauce.

# *PICKLE CHIPS*

**Preparation Time:** 15 minutes

**Cooking Time:** 22 minutes

**Servings:** 6

## Nutritional values:

- Calories: 177 kcal
- Fat: 9.1 g
- Carbohydrates: 18.6 g
- Proteins: 5.6 g

## Ingredients:

- 2 large eggs
- 1 tsp. lemon juice
- 1 tbsp. Creole mustard
- 1 reduced-sodium dill pickle chips jar
- 1 cup panko breadcrumbs
- ½ tsp. smoked paprika
- ½ cup all-purpose flour
- ¼ cup mayonnaise

## Directions:

1. Beat the eggs in a small bowl lightly.

2. Pour the flour into another bowl and place the panko in a third bowl.

3. Drain the pickle chips before patting them dry with paper towels.

4. Now, soak the pickle chips in the flour and shake off excess. Just ensure that they are well coated.

5. After dipping the in flour, you need to dip them in the beaten eggs. Now, you can toss the coated pickles in panko.

6. Divide the pickles into three batches so that you can air fry them batch by batch.

7. Cook the first batch at 350°F for 6 minutes. They should be tender, crispy, and golden brown by then.

8. Do the same to the remaining two batches.

9. Mix the smoked paprika, lemon juice, Creole mustard, and mayonnaise together in another bowl. Serve the pickle chips with the mayonnaise mixture as dipping sauce.

# *CHICKPEAS*

**Preparation Time:** 15 minutes

**Cooking Time:** 18 minutes

**Servings:** 4

**Nutritional values:**

- Calories: 80 kcal
- Fat: 1.5 g
- Carbohydrates: 13 g
- Proteins: 4 g

**Ingredients:**

- Non-stick cooking spray
- 1/8 tsp. cayenne, or to taste
- 1 can no-salt-added chickpeas (it should be drained and rinsed)
- ½ tsp. garlic powder
- ½ tsp. coarse ground black pepper
- ½ tsp. dried thyme leaves

## Directions:

1. Pour the chickpea into a bowl and pat it dry with paper towels. The next step is to spray the cooking spray on the chickpeas.

2. Toss it to make it evenly coated.

3. Now, you can pour the chickpeas into your air fryer basket.

4. Mix cayenne, pepper, thyme leaves, and garlic powder together.

5. Air fry the chickpeas for about 15 minutes at 375°F. You should keep shaking and checking it every 5 minutes because it may get crispy and done in less than 15 minutes.

6. You may also spray a little cooking spray on it while it is being cooked.

7. When it is done, pour it in a bowl and season it. We will advise you to season it when it is still hot to boost the adherence of the seasoning.

8. You can now allow it to cool further or serve it warm. To preserve it, you need to store it in an airtight container.

# *WATER SPINACH*

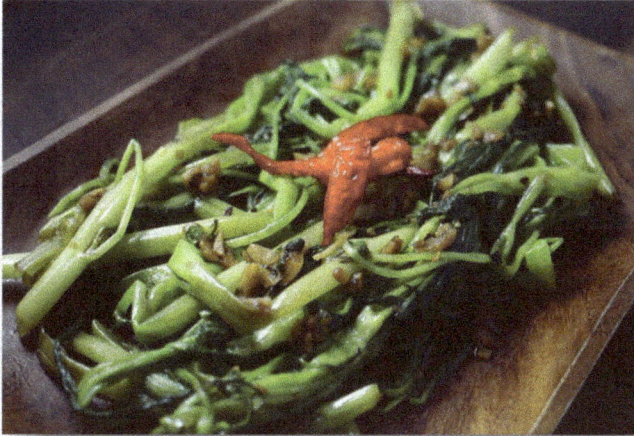

**Preparation Time:** 8 minutes

**Cooking Time:** 2 minutes

**Servings:** 4

## Nutritional values:

- Calories: 19
- Fat: 0.2 g
- Carbohydrates: 3.1 g
- Proteins: 2.6 g

## Ingredients:

- 2½ pounds fresh water spinach
- Pinch sea salt, to taste

## Directions:

1. Preheat Air Fryer to 330°F.
2. Put water spinach in the Air fryer basket. Fry for 20 seconds. Drain on paper towels. Repeat the step with the rest of the water spinach. Season with salt. Serve.

# LEAN BEEF DUMPLINGS

**Preparation Time:** 9 minutes

**Cooking Time:** 27 minutes

**Servings:** 3

## Nutritional values:

- Calories: 77
- Fat: 3.5 g
- Carbohydrates: 7.5 g
- Proteins: 3.2 g

## Ingredients:

- 12 pieces circular gyoza, thick, large

Filling:

- ½ cup lean ground beef
- ¼ cup loosely Napa cabbage, julienned
- 1/8 Tsp. fresh ginger, grated
- 1 garlic clove, grated
- ¼ tsp. miso paste

- ¼ Tbsp. green onions, roots trimmed, minced
- ¼ tsp. sesame oil
- 1/8 tsp. kosher salt
- 1/16 tsp. white sugar

Sauce:

- 2 tbsp. dark soy sauce
- 1/16 tsp. chili oil
- 1 tbsp. rice vinegar

## Directions:

1. Preheat the Air Fryer to 400°F.
2. Meanwhile, combine all filling ingredients in a bowl.
3. Place a dumpling/gyoza wrapper on a flat surface. Scoop in ½ tsp. of the filling.
4. Moisten edges of wrapper with water. Fold wrapper into two. Seal edges well. Pleat edges. You have the option to do this or not.
5. Hold on to the edges of the dumpling and gently tap bottoms on a flat surface to make the base even. Repeat step for all fillings and wrappers. Place on a baking sheet lined with parchment paper. Freeze for an hour before frying.
6. To make the sauce, mix the ingredients in a small bowl. Set aside until needed.

7.      Place six frozen gyoza into the air fryer basket. Place double layer rack on top, and add in more dumplings, making sure none overlap.

8.      Cook for 12 minutes, or until wrappers turn golden brown. Remove and place on plates. Loosely tent with aluminum foil—repeat step for all dumplings.

9.      Serve equal portions on plates, with a small amount of sauce on the side.

# *ALL HERBS AND CHEESE CHICKEN*

**Preparation Time:** 8 minutes

**Cooking Time:** 26 minutes

**Servings:** 4

## Nutritional values:

- Calories: 180
- Fat: 3.5 g
- Carbohydrates: 20 g
- Proteins: 18 g

## Ingredients:

- 4 chicken breasts, skinless, boneless, halved
- 2 tsp. tarragon, chopped
- 1 tbsp. parsley, chopped
- 1 tbsp. dill, chopped
- ½ goat cheese, crumbled, reduced-fat
- 3 tbsp. basil, chopped

- 2 tsp. lemon zest, grated
- ½ tsp. salt
- ¼ tsp. pepper

**Directions:**

1. Preheat the Air Fryer to 350°F.
2. Coat herbed chicken with little cooking oil.
3. In a bowl, combine lemon zest, tarragon, parsley, dill, and basil. Add goat cheese into the mixture. Set aside some of the herb mixtures.
4. Make a small pocket in the chicken breast. Each pocket should be filled with the herb mixture. Secure pocket using a toothpick. Season with salt, pepper, and herb mixture.
5. Cook chicken for 10 minutes on each side. Serve.

# *LEAN PORK AND SHRIMP DUMPLINGS*

**Preparation Time:** 9 minutes

**Cooking Time:** 21 minutes

**Servings:** 4

## Nutritional values:

- Calories: 180
- Fat: 6 g
- Carbohydrates: 20 g
- Proteins: 10 g

## Ingredients:

- 12 thin wonton wrappers, separated

Filling:

- ½ cup lean ground pork
- ½ cup peeled shrimps, uncooked, chopped
- 1/8 cup carrots, diced

- 1/8 cup jicama, diced
- 1/8 cup chives, chopped roughly
- 1/8 tsp. rice wine
- 1/8 tsp. sea salt
- 1/16 tsp. black pepper

Sauce:

- 2 tbsp. light soy sauce
- 1 tbsp. lime juice, freshly squeezed
- ¼ tsp. roasted sesame oil
- 1/8 tsp. stevia

**Directions:**

1. Preheat the Air Fryer to 300°F.
2. To make dumplings, combine filling ingredients in a food processor. Process until the mixture looks like a coarse paste. Rest for 5 minutes before wrapping.
3. Drape dumpling wrapper. Scoop in ½ tbsp. of filling. Moisten edges of wrapper with water.
4. Gently press down on filling until the dumpling gently slides between your fingers and into your palm. Squeeze in dumpling sides, but leave the top open. Gently tap dumplings on a flat surface to make the base even. Continue pinching and tapping until the dumpling can stand on its own. Place on a baking sheet lined with

parchment paper. Repeat step for all fillings and wrappers. Freeze for at least ½ hour before frying. Do not thaw.

5. Place into the Air Fryer basket. Cook for 15 minutes, or until wrappers turn golden brown and tops are set. Remove from the basket.

6. For the sauce: pour ingredients in a bowl. Stir until sugar dissolves.

7. Serve equal portions on plates with a small amount of sauce on the side.

# *CHICKEN AND MUSHROOMS IN COCONUT CREAM*

**Preparation Time:** 5 minutes

**Cooking Time:** 28 minutes

**Servings:** 4

## Nutritional values:

- Calories: 174 kcal
- Fat: 4.5 g
- Carbohydrates: 8.4 g
- Proteins: 24.1 g

## Ingredients:

- 1 can button mushrooms, rinsed well; large caps halved/quartered
- 1½ cups cooked Basmati rice
- 1/8 cup fresh cilantro, minced

Chicken and marinade:

- 4 chicken thigh fillets, cubed
- ½ tbsp. fresh ginger, peeled, grated
- 1 piece bird's eye chili, minced, optional
- 1 can thick coconut cream
- 1 tbsp. fresh lemongrass bulb, tough parts peeled off, minced
- 1/16 tsp. salt
- 1/16 tsp. white pepper

**Directions:**

1. Preheat the Air Fryer to 355°F. Cook dish for 5 minutes.
2. Combine chicken and marinade in a large bowl. Set aside in the fridge for at least 30 minutes to steep. Divide into 2 equal portions.
3. To prepare the tiffin box, spread cooked rice evenly into the bottom of the tiffin box. Sprinkle mushrooms evenly on top.
4. Pour chicken and marinade on top of mushrooms. Seal lid. Set this aside for 10 minutes, or until the chicken comes to room temperature.
5. Place sealed tiffin box into Air Fryer basket.
6. Turn down heat to 285°F. Continue cooking for another 15 minutes. Turn off the machine immediately. Leave the tiffin box in the basket for 5 minutes to rest.
7. Remove tiffin box. Carefully take off the lid. Garnish the dish with cilantro. Serve right out of tiffin box

# *BEEF TENDERLOIN WITH VEGETABLES*

**Preparation Time:** 8 minutes

**Cooking Time:** 23 minutes

**Servings:** 4

## Nutritional values:

- Calories: 89.4 kcal
- Fat: 3.5 g
- Carbohydrates: 0.5 g
- Proteins: 13.2 g

## Ingredients:

- 2½ pounds beef tenderloin
- ½ green bell pepper, julienned
- ½ red bell pepper, deseeded, ribbed, julienned
- 2 tbsp. light soy sauce
- 1 cup almond flour, finely milled
- ¼ tsp. black pepper

- Pinch stevia
- Pinch sea salt
- 3 tbsp. olive oil
- 2 onions, julienned
- 1 banana chili, julienned
- Pinch sea salt
- Pinch black pepper

## Directions:

1. Preheat Air Fryer to 330°F.
2. Put beef tenderloin in a food-safe bag together with the marinade ingredients. Massage beef and shake well. Put inside the refrigerator for 1 hour or overnight.
3. Layer beef in the air fryer basket. Fry for 5 minutes on each side or until beef is lightly brown in color. Repeat step until all meat is cooked.
4. Meanwhile, sauté peppers and onion in a pan for 2 minutes. Spoon veggies on a plate. Serve with beef tenderloin.

# *BUTTER-LEMON CHICKEN*

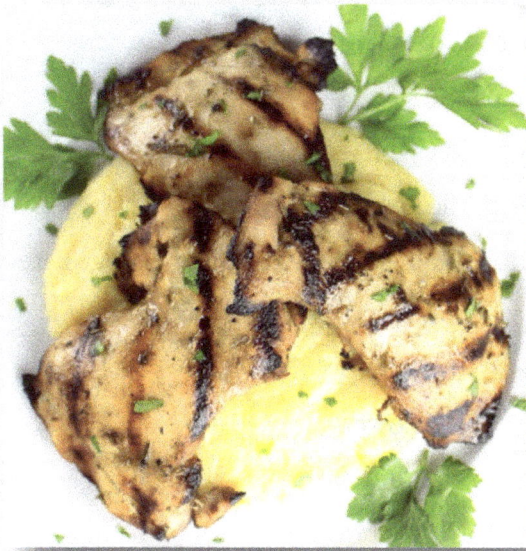

**Preparation Time:** 6 minutes

**Cooking Time:** 60 minutes

**Servings:** 3

**Nutritional values:**

- Calories: 260
- Fat: 14.5 g
- Carbohydrates: 2.0 g
- Proteins: 54.9 g

## Ingredients:

- 4 pieces corn on the cob, halved into equal portions
- ¼ tbsp. butter
- 1/16 tsp. fine salt
- 1 5 to 5.6 lbs. whole chicken, skinless
- 1 large garlic head, keep whole
- 1 lemon, half sliced into equal wedges, remaining half squeezed but reserve spent lemon rind
- ½ tbsp. smoky paprika powder
- ¼ tsp. garlic powder
- 2 tbsp. butter, low-fat
- ¼ tsp. turmeric powder
- ¼ tsp. onion powder
- 1/8 tsp. stevia
- 1 tbsp. salt
- 1/8 tsp. black pepper
- 2 tbsp. olive oil

## Directions:

1. Preheat the Air Fryer to 360°F.
2. Find a spot under the chicken breast where skin and meat can be gently separated. Using your fingers, rub butter under the skin, right up to the creases.

3.    In a bowl, mix together black pepper, stevia, garlic powder, kosher salt, olive oil, onion powder, paprika powder, and turmeric powder. Rub mixture vigorously all over the chicken, including inside the cavity.

4.    Stuff garlic and spent lemon rind inside the chicken.

5.    Place chicken, breast side down into Air Fryer basket. Cook for 60 minutes. Flip chicken right side up midway through cooking.

6.    Remove chicken from the basket. Place on a platter. Drizzle in half of the lemon juice.

7.    Loosely tent chicken with sheet of aluminum foil. Rest for at least 10 minutes before discarding garlic head and lemon rind. Carve into desired pieces.

8.    Drizzle in remaining lemon juice.

9.    For the corn, rub butter all over the corn. Wrap each piece individually in sheets of aluminum foil.

10.   Place these in the air Fryer basket, still at the same heat setting. Cook for 6 minutes.

11.   Remove corn from basket. Cool slightly before removing the aluminum foil. Season corn with a small amount of salt just before serving.

12.   Serve the desired amount of chicken with a corn on the side.

# *DOUBLE-GLAZED AIR-FRIED CINNAMON BISCUIT BITES*

**Preparation Time:** 9 minutes

**Cooking Time:** 28 minutes

**Servings:** 8

**Nutritional values:**

- Calories: 325 kcal
- Fat: 7 g
- Carbohydrates: 60 g
- Proteins: 8 g

**Ingredients:**

- 2/3 cup whole-wheat flour
- 2/3 cup all-purpose flour
- 1 tsp. baking powder
- 2 tbsp. granulated sugar
- ¼ tsp. kosher salt

- ¼ tsp. ground cinnamon
- 4 tbsp. cold salted butter
- 1/3 cup whole milk
- Cooking spray
- 3 tbsp. water
- 2 cups powdered sugar

## Directions:

1. Cut salted butter into small pieces, set aside.
2. Whisk in a medium bowl the whole-wheat and all-purpose flours, baking powder, granulated sugar, salt, and cinnamon.
3. Add the butter pieces and with a pastry cutter, cut into the flour mixture until well blended and looks like a coarse cornmeal.
4. Stir in milk until the dough forms into a ball. Lay the dough on a floured work surface. Knead for thirty seconds until smooth and forms into a solid ball.
5. With a pastry cutter, cut the dough into sixteen equal portions; roll into a smooth ball.
6. Mist the air fryer basket with cooking spray. Arrange the first half of the balls in the basket, with at least 1 inch apart. Spray the donut balls with cooking spray; cook for ten to 12 minutes at 350°F until puffed and browned.

7.  Slowly remove the balls from the basket and transfer to a wire rack, slightly covered with foil. Repeat with the remaining half of the donut balls. Let cool for five minutes.

8.  Prepare the glaze by whisking together in a bowl the powdered sugar and water until smooth.

9.  Spoon half of the glaze all over the donut balls. Let cool for 5 minutes and glaze again and let drip naturally into a bowl.

10. Serve!

# *AIR-FRIED APPLE CHIPS*

**Preparation Time:** 14 minutes

**Cooking Time:** 22 minutes

**Servings:** 4

## Nutritional values:

- Calories: 104
- Fat: 3 g
- Carbohydrates: 17 g
- Proteins: 1 g

## Ingredients:

- 1 (8 ounces) Fuji or Honey crisp apple
- 2 tsp. canola oil
- 1 tsp. ground cinnamon
- Cooking spray
- 1 tbsp. almond butter
- ¼ cup plain 1% low-fat Greek yogurt
- 1 tsp. honey

## Directions:

1. Using a mandolin, thinly slice the apple and place it in a bowl with oil and cinnamon. Toss the apples to evenly coat.

2. Spray the air fryer with a light coating of cooking spray.

3. Arrange seven to eight slices of apples in a single layer in the basket. Cook for twelve minutes at 375°F, turning every four minutes, and then rearrange the slices with a wooden ladle to flatten them as they tend to curl during cooking.

4. Repeat with the remaining apple slices. Let cool until crisp, naturally.

5. Combine in a small bowl the almond butter, honey, and yogurt, stirring until smooth.

6. Arrange six to eight apple slices on an individual plate and serve with a small dollop of the honey-butter-yogurt dipping sauce.

7. Serve!

# AIR FRYER EMPANADAS

**Preparation Time:** 11 minutes

**Cooking Time:** 29 minutes

**Servings:** 2

**Nutritional values:**

- Calories: 343 kcal
- Fat: 19 g
- Carbohydrates: 25 g
- Proteins: 17 g

**Ingredients:**

- 1 tbsp. olive oil
- ¼ cup finely chopped white onion
- 3 ounces (85/15) lean ground beef
- 3 ounces finely chopped cremini mushrooms
- 2 tsp. finely chopped garlic
- ¼ tsp. paprika
- 6 chopped pitted green olives
- 1/8 tsp. ground cinnamon

- ¼ tsp. ground cumin
- ½ cup chopped tomatoes
- 8 pieces square gyoza wrappers
- 1 lightly beaten large egg

## Directions:

1. Heat the olive oil in a medium skillet over medium-high.
2. Add the onion and beef; cook and stir using a wooden spoon until crumbly and starts to brown for 3 minutes.
3. Sauté the cremini mushrooms. Stir and cook for six minutes until it starts to brown. Sauté the garlic and olives; stir in cinnamon and cumin. Continue cooking for three more minutes until the mushrooms have released their liquid and very tender.
4. Add the tomatoes, stir for 1 minute. Pour the filling into a large bowl, let cool for five minutes.
5. Place four pieces of gyoza wrappers on a work surface and fill the center with 1 ½ tbsp. of meat filling.
6. To seal, brush the edges of gyoza wrappers with egg, fold over and pinch. Follow these steps for the rest of the filling and wrappers.
7. Arrange four empanadas in an air fryer basket in one layer. Cook at 400°F for seven minutes until evenly browned. Cook the remaining empanadas.

# AIR-FRIED CALZONES

**Preparation Time:** 9 minutes

**Cooking Time:** 26 minutes

**Servings:** 2

## Nutritional values:

- Calories: 348 kcal
- Fat: 12 g
- Carbohydrates: 44 g
- Proteins: 21 g

## Ingredients:

- 1 tsp. olive oil
- ¼ cup finely chopped red onion
- 3 ounces baby spinach leaves
- 2 ounces shredded rotisserie chicken breast
- 1/3 cup lower-sodium marinara sauce
- 6 ounces fresh prepared whole-wheat pizza dough
- 1 ½ ounces pre-shredded part-skim mozzarella cheese
- Cooking spray

## Directions:

1. Heat the olive oil in a medium nonstick pan on medium-high.
2. Stir-fry the onion in hot oil for two minutes until tender and fragrant.
3. Sauté the spinach and then cover and cook for 1 ½ minute until wilted. Remove the pan from heat.
4. Pour the marinara sauce and shredded chicken into the pan, stir to combine.
5. Divide the whole-wheat pizza dough into four equal sizes; roll into a six" circle on a lightly floured work surface.
6. Fill about ¼ of the spinach filling on top of the individual dough circle. Spread on top of spinach with ¼ of mozzarella cheese.
7. Create half-moons by folding the dough over the filling and crimp the edges to seal.
8. Before placing the calzones in the air fryer basket, coat them with a generous amount of cooking spray. Cook at 325°F for 12 minutes, until golden brown.
9. Turn the calzones over after eight minutes of cooking.
10. Serve!

# *AIR-FRIED BEET CHIPS*

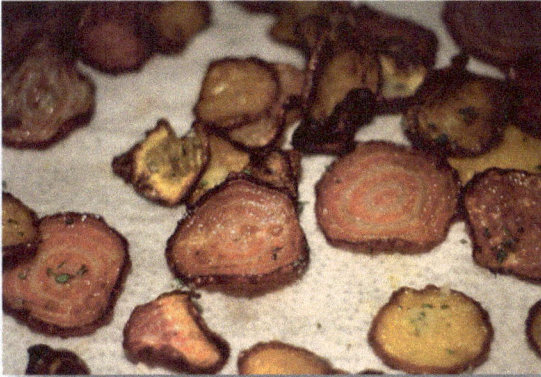

**Preparation Time:** 9 minutes

**Cooking Time:** 25-30 minutes

**Servings:** 4

**Nutritional values:**

- Calories: 47 kcal
- Fat: 2 g
- Carbohydrates: 6 g
- Proteins: 1 g

**Ingredients:**

- 2 tsp. canola oil

- 3 medium-size red beets
- ¼ tsp. black pepper
- 3/4 tsp. kosher salt

## Directions:

1. Peel the red beets and cut into 1/8" thick slices, yields about 3 cups of slices.

2. Mix together in a large bowl the oil, pepper, and salt and toss the sliced beets to coat well.

3. Arrange half of the red beets in the basket of your air fryer.

4. Cook at 320°F for twenty-five to thirty minutes until crisp and totally dry.

5. Shake the basket every five minutes. Repeat the same steps for the rest of the beets.

# AIR FRYER SWEET POTATO CHIPS

**Preparation Time:** 13 minutes

**Cooking Time:** 28 minutes

**Servings:** 4

## Nutritional values:

- Calories: 60 kcal
- Fat: 3.5 g
- Carbohydrates: 7 g
- Proteins: 1 g

## Ingredients:

- 1 medium unpeeled sweet potato, cut into 1/8-inch-thick slices
- ¼ tsp. sea salt
- 1 tbsp. canola oil
- ¼ tsp. freshly ground black pepper

- 1 tsp. chopped fresh rosemary (optional)
- Cooking spray

## Directions:

1. Fill a large bowl with cold water. Soak the sweet potato slices in cold water for twenty minutes. Drain in colander and pat dry with paper towels.

2. Dry the bowl and use it to mix the canola oil, pepper, salt, and optional chopped fresh rosemary.

3. Add the sweet potatoes and gently toss until well coated.

4. Mist lightly with cooking spray the air fryer basket and place inside half of the sweet potatoes.

5. Cook in batches of two at 350°F for fifteen minutes until crispy and thoroughly cooked.

6. Transfer the chips to a large plate, let cool, and serve warm. You can store the remaining chips in a sealed plastic container for your next snacks.

# *HERBED PORK RIBS*

**Preparation Time:** 6 minutes

**Cooking Time:** 20-25 minutes

**Servings:** 4

## Nutritional values:

- Calories: 296 kcal
- Fat: 3.41 g
- Carbohydrates: 6 g
- Proteins: 29 g

## Ingredients:

- 500g pork ribs
- Provencal herbs
- Salt
- Ground pepper
- Oil

## Directions:

1. Put the ribs in a bowl and add some oil, Provencal herbs, salt, and ground pepper.
2. Stir well and leave in the fridge for at least 1 hour.
3. Put the ribs in the basket of the air fryer and select 200°C, 20 minutes.
4. From time to time, shake the basket and remove the ribs.

# MUSTARD LAMB LOIN CHOPS

**Preparation Time:** 15 minutes

**Cooking Time:** 30 minutes

**Servings:** 4

## Nutritional values:

- Calories: 433 kcal
- Fat: 17.6 g
- Carbohydrates: 0.6 g
- Proteins: 64.1 g

## Ingredients:

- 8: 4-ounces lamb loin chops
- 2 tbsp. Dijon mustard
- 1 tbsp. fresh lemon juice
- ½ tsp. olive oil
- 1 tsp. dried tarragon
- Salt and black pepper, to taste

## Directions:

1. Preheat the Air fryer to 390°F and grease an Air fryer basket.
2. Mix the mustard, lemon juice, oil, tarragon, salt, and black pepper in a large bowl.
3. Coat the chops generously with the mustard mixture and arrange them in the air fryer basket.
4. Cook for about 15 minutes, flipping once in between, and dish out to serve hot.

# *HERBED LAMB CHOPS*

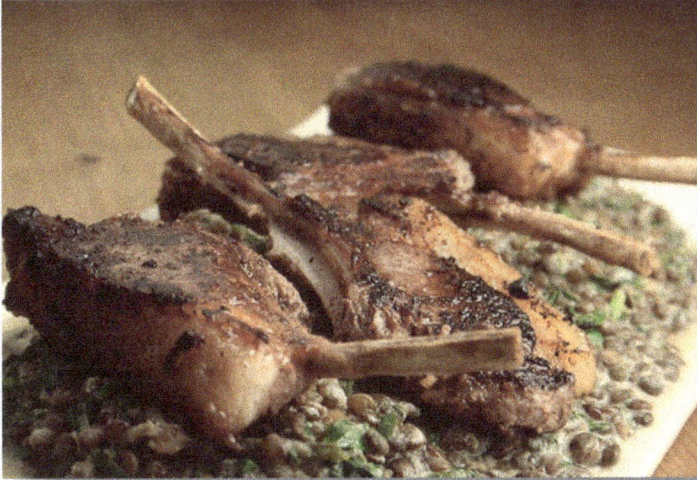

**Preparation Time:** 10 minutes

**Cooking Time:** 7 minutes

**Servings:** 2

**Nutritional values:**

- Calories: 491 kcal
- Fat: 24 g
- Carbohydrates: 1.6 g
- Proteins: 64 g

## Ingredients:

- 4: 4-ounces lamb chops
- 1 tbsp. fresh lemon juice
- 1 tbsp. olive oil
- 1 tsp. dried rosemary
- 1 tsp. dried thyme
- 1 tsp. dried oregano
- ½ tsp. ground cumin
- ½ tsp. ground coriander
- Salt and black pepper, to taste

## Directions:

1. Preheat the Air fryer to 390°F and grease an Air fryer basket.
2. Mix the lemon juice, oil, herbs, and spices in a large bowl.
3. Coat the chops generously with the herb mixture and refrigerate to marinate for about 1 hour.
4. Arrange the chops in the Air fryer basket and cook for about 7 minutes, flipping once in between.
5. Dish out the lamb chops in a platter and serve hot.

# ZAATAR LAMB LOIN CHOPS

**Preparation Time:** 10 minutes

**Cooking Time:** 15-20 minutes

**Servings:** 4

## Nutritional values:

- Calories: 433 kcal
- Fat: 17.6 g
- Carbohydrates: 0.6 g
- Proteins: 64.1 g

## Ingredients:

- 8: 3½-ounces bone-in lamb loin chops, trimmed
- 3 garlic cloves, crushed
- 1 tbsp. fresh lemon juice
- 1 tsp. olive oil
- 1 tbsp. Zaatar
- Salt and black pepper, to taste

## Directions:

1. Preheat the Air fryer to 400°F and grease an Air fryer basket.
2. Mix the garlic, lemon juice, oil, Zaatar, salt, and black pepper in a large bowl.
3. Coat the chops generously with the herb mixture and arrange the chops in the air fryer basket.
4. Cook for about 15 minutes, flipping twice in between, and dish out the lamb chops to serve hot.

# PESTO COATED RACK OF LAMB

**Preparation Time:** 15 minutes

**Cooking Time:** 15 minutes

**Servings:** 4

## Nutritional values:

- Calories: 406 kcal
- Fat: 27.7 g
- Carbohydrates: 2.9 g
- Proteins: 34.9 g

## Ingredients:

- ½ bunch fresh mint
- 1: 1½-pounds rack of lamb
- 1 garlic clove
- ¼ cup extra-virgin olive oil
- ½ tbsp. honey
- Salt and black pepper, to taste

## Directions:

1.  Preheat the Air fryer to 200|F and grease an Air fryer basket.
2.  Put the mint, garlic, oil, honey, salt, and black pepper in a blender and pulse until smooth to make pesto.
3.  Coat the rack of lamb with this pesto on both sides and arrange it in the air fryer basket.
4.  Cook for about 15 minutes and cut the rack into individual chops to serve.

# SPICED LAMB STEAKS

**Preparation Time:** 15 minutes

**Cooking Time:** 15 minutes

**Servings:** 3

## Nutritional values:

- Calories: 252 kcal
- Fat: 16.7 g
- Carbohydrates: 4.2 g
- Proteins: 21.7 g

## Ingredients:

- ½ onion, roughly chopped
- 1½ pounds boneless lamb sirloin steaks
- 5 garlic cloves, peeled
- 1 tbsp. fresh ginger, peeled
- 1 tsp. garam masala
- 1 tsp. ground fennel
- ½ tsp. ground cumin
- ½ tsp. ground cinnamon

- ½ tsp. cayenne pepper
- Salt and black pepper, to taste

## Directions:

1. Preheat the Air fryer to 330°F and grease an Air fryer basket.
2. Put the onion, garlic, ginger, and spices in a blender and pulse until smooth.
3. Coat the lamb steaks with this mixture on both sides and refrigerate to marinate for about 24 hours.
4. Arrange the lamb steaks in the air fryer basket and cook for about 15 minutes, flipping once in between.
5. Dish out the steaks in a platter and serve warm.

# *AIR FRYER SHRIMP SCAMPI*

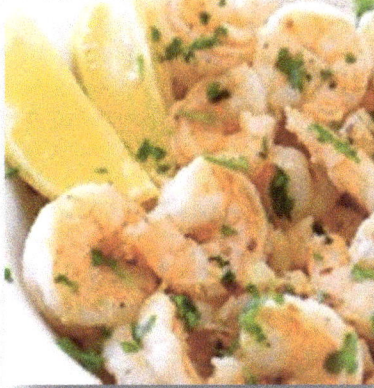

**Preparation Time:** 5 minutes

**Cooking Time:** 11 minutes

**Servings:** 2

**Nutritional values:**

- Calories: 287 kcal
- Fat: 5.5 g
- Carbohydrates: 7.5 g
- Proteins: 18 g

## Ingredients:

- 4 cups raw shrimp
- 1 tbsp. lemon juice
- Chopped fresh basil
- 2 tsp. red pepper flakes
- 2.5 tbsp. butter
- Chopped chives
- 2 tbsp. chicken stock
- 1 tbsp. minced garlic

## Directions:

1. Let the air fryer preheat with a metal pan to 330°F
2. In the hot pan, add garlic, red pepper flakes, and half of the butter. Let it cook for two minutes.
3. Add the butter, shrimp, chicken stock, minced garlic, chives, lemon juice, and basil to the pan. Let it cook for five minutes. Bathe the shrimp in melted butter.
4. Take out from the air fryer and let it rest for one minute.
5. Add fresh basil leaves and chives and serve.

# *SESAME SEEDS FISH FILLET*

**Preparation Time:** 11 minutes

**Cooking Time:** 15 minutes

**Servings:** 2

## Nutritional values:

- Calories: 250 kcal
- Fat: 8 g
- Carbohydrates: 12.4 g
- Proteins: 20 g

## Ingredients:

- 3 tbsp. plain flour
- 1 egg, beaten
- 5 frozen fish fillets

For Coating:

- 2 tbsp. oil
- ½ cup Sesame seeds
- Rosemary herbs

- 5-6 biscuit's crumbs
- Kosher salt and pepper, to taste

## Directions:

1. For two-minute sauté the sesame seeds in a pan, without oil. Brown them and set it aside.
2. On a plate, mix all coating ingredients
3. Place the aluminum foil on the air fryer basket and let it preheat at 200°C.
4. First, coat the fish in flour. Then in egg, then in the coating mix.
5. Place in the Air fryer. If fillets are frozen, cook for ten minutes, then turn the fillet and cook for another four minutes.
6. If not frozen, then cook for eight minutes and two minutes.

# *LEMON PEPPER SHRIMP IN AIR FRYER*

**Preparation Time:** 5 minutes

**Cooking Time:** 11 minutes

**Servings:** 2

## Nutritional values:

- Calories: 237 kcal
- Fat: 6 g
- Carbohydrates: 11 g
- Proteins: 36 g

## Ingredients:

- 1 and ½ raw shrimp, cup peeled, deveined
- ½ tbsp. olive oil
- ¼ tsp. garlic powder
- 1 tsp. lemon pepper
- ¼ tsp. paprika
- 1 lemon, juiced

## Directions:

1. Let the air fryer preheat to 400°F
2. In a bowl, mix lemon pepper, olive oil, paprika, garlic powder, and lemon juice. Mix well. Add shrimps and coat well
3. Add shrimps in the air fryer, cook for 6 to 8 minutes and top with lemon slices and serve

# *SOUTHWEST CHICKEN IN AIR FRYER*

**Preparation Time:** 20 minutes

**Cooking Time:** 30 minutes

**Servings:** 4

## Nutritional values:

- Calories: 165 kcal
- Fat: 6 g
- Carbohydrates: 1 g
- Proteins: 24 g

## Ingredients:

- Avocado oil: one tbsp.
- Four cups boneless, skinless, chicken breast
- Chili powder: half tsp.

- Salt to taste
- Cumin: half tsp.
- Onion powder: ¼ tsp.
- Lime juice: two tbsp.
- Garlic powder: ¼ tsp.

## Directions:

1. In a Ziplock bag, add chicken, oil, and lime juice.
2. Add all spices in a bowl and rub all over the chicken in the Ziplock bag.
3. Let it marinate in the fridge for ten minutes or more.
4. Take chicken out from the Ziplock bag and put it in the air fryer.
5. Cook for 25 minutes at 400°F, flipping chicken halfway through until internal temperature reaches 165°F.

# NO-BREADING CHICKEN BREAST IN AIR FRYER

**Preparation Time:** 10 minutes

**Cooking Time:** 20 minutes

**Servings:** 2

## Nutritional values:

- Calories: 208 kcal
- Fat: 4.5 g
- Carbohydrates: 1 g
- Proteins: 39 g

## Ingredients:

- Olive oil spray
- 4 (boneless) chicken breasts
- ¾ tsp. onion powder
- ¼ cup salt:
- 1/2 tsp. smoked paprika
- 1/8 tsp. cayenne pepper

- ¾ tsp. garlic powder
- ½ tsp. dried parsley

## Directions:

1. In a large bowl, add six cups of warm water, add salt (¼ cup), and mix to dissolve.
2. Put chicken breasts in the warm salted water and let it refrigerate for almost 2 hours.
3. Remove from water and pat dry.
4. In a bowl, add all the spices with ¾ tsp. of salt. Spray the oil all over the chicken and rub the spice mix all over the chicken.
5. Let the air fryer heat at 380F.
6. Put the chicken in the air fryer and cook for ten minutes. Flip halfway through and serve with salad green.

# *LEMON PEPPER CHICKEN BREAST*

**Preparation Time:** 3 minutes

**Cooking Time:** 15 minutes

**Servings:** 2

## Nutritional values:

- Calories: 140 kcal
- Fat: 2 g
- Carbohydrates: 24 g
- Proteins: 13 g

## Ingredients:

- Two Lemons rind, juice, and zest
- 1 chicken breast
- 1 tsp. minced garlic
- 2 tbsp. black peppercorns
- 1 tbsp. chicken seasoning
- Salt & pepper, to taste

## Directions:

1. Let the air fryer preheat to 180°C.
2. In a large aluminum foil, add all the seasonings along with lemon rind.
3. Add salt and pepper to the chicken and rub the seasonings all over the chicken breast.
4. Put the chicken in aluminum foil. And fold it tightly.
5. Flatten the chicken inside foil with a rolling pin
6. Put it in the air fryer and cook at 180°C for 15 minutes.
7. Serve hot.

# *HERB-MARINATED CHICKEN THIGHS*

**Preparation Time:** 30 minutes

**Cooking Time:** 12-15 minutes

**Servings:** 4

## Nutritional values:

- Calories: 100 kcal
- Fat: 9 g
- Carbohydrates: 1 g
- Proteins 4 g

## Ingredients:

- 8 chicken thighs, skin-on, bone-in
- 2 tbsp. lemon juice
- 1/2 tsp. onion powder
- 2 tsp. garlic powder
- 1 tsp. spike seasoning
- ¼ cup olive oil

- 1 tsp. dried basil
- 1/2 tsp. dried oregano
- ¼ tsp. black pepper

## Directions:

1. In a bowl, add dried oregano, olive oil, lemon juice, dried sage, garlic powder, Spike Seasoning, onion powder, dried basil, black pepper.
2. In a Ziplock bag, add the spice blend and the chicken and mix well.
3. Marinate the chicken in the refrigerator for at least six hours or more.
4. Preheat the air fryer to 360°F.
5. Put the chicken in the air fryer basket, cook for six-eight minutes, flip the chicken, and cook for six minutes more.
6. Until the internal chicken temperature reaches 165°F.
7. Take out from the air fryer and serve.

# AIR FRIED CHICKEN FAJITAS

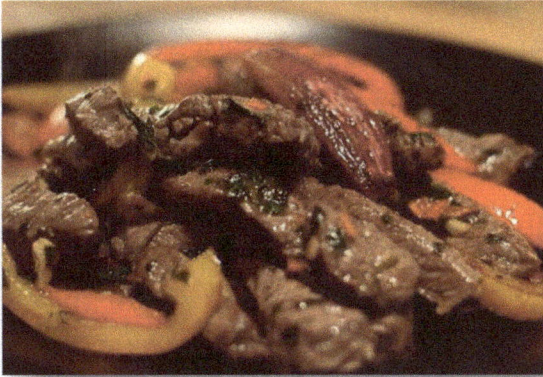

**Preparation Time:** 10 minutes

**Cooking Time:** 20 minutes

**Servings:** 6

## Nutritional values:

- Calories: 140 kcal
- Fat: 5 g
- Proteins: 22 g
- Carbohydrates: 6g

## Ingredients:

- 4 cups, cut into thin strips chicken breasts
- Bell peppers, sliced
- 1/2 tsp. salt
- 1 tsp. cumin
- ¼ tsp. garlic powder
- 1/2 tsp. chili powder
- 1 tbsp. lime juice

## Directions:

1. In a bowl, add seasonings, chicken, and lime juice, and mix well.
2. Then add sliced peppers and coat well.
3. Spray the air fryer with olive oil.
4. Put the chicken and peppers in, and cook for 15 minutes at 400°F. flip halfway through.
5. Serve with wedges of lemons and enjoy.

# *BLACKENED CHICKEN BREAST*

**Preparation Time:** 10 minutes

**Cooking Time:** 20 minutes

**Servings:** 2

## Nutritional values:

- Calories: 432.1 kcal
- Fat: 9.5 g
- Carbohydrates: 3.2 g
- Proteins: 79.4 g

## Ingredients:

- 2 tsp. paprika
- 1 tsp. ground thyme
- 1 tsp. cumin
- 1/2 tsp. cayenne pepper
- 1/2 tsp. onion powder
- 1/2 tsp. black pepper

- ¼ tsp. salt:
- 2 tsp. vegetable oil
- Pieces chicken breast halves (without bones and skin)

## Directions:

1. In a mixing bowl, add onion powder, salt, cumin, paprika, black pepper, thyme, and cayenne pepper. Mix it well.
2. Drizzle oil over chicken and rub. Dip each piece of chicken in a blackening spice blend on both sides.
3. Let it rest for five minutes while the air fryer is preheating.
4. Preheat it for five minutes at 360°F.
5. Put the chicken in the air fryer and let it cook for ten minutes. Flip and then cook for another ten minutes.
6. After, let it sit for five minutes, then slice and serve with the side of greens.

# CHICKEN WITH MIXED VEGETABLES

**Preparation Time:** 20 minutes

**Cooking Time:** 20 minutes

**Servings:** 2

## Nutritional values:

- Calories: 230 kcal
- Fat: 10 g
- Carbohydrates: 8 g
- Proteins: 26 g

## Ingredients:

- ½ onion diced
- 4 cups, cubed pieces chicken breast
- 1/2 zucchini chopped
- 1 tbsp. Italian seasoning
- ½ cup bell pepper, chopped
- 2 cloves of garlic, pressed

- ½ cup broccoli florets
- 2 tbsp. olive oil
- 1/2 tsp. chili powder, garlic powder, pepper, salt

## Directions:

1. Let the air fryer heat to 400°F and dice the vegetables
2. In a bowl, add the seasoning, oil, and add vegetables, chicken and toss well
3. Place chicken and vegetables in the air fryer, and cook for ten minutes, toss halfway through, cook in batches.
4. Make sure the veggies are charred, and the chicken is cooked through.
5. Serve hot.

# *CAULIFLOWER FLORETS AND SWEET POTATO PATTIES*

**Preparation Time:** 9 minutes

**Cooking Time:** 39 minutes

**Servings:** 7

**Nutritional values:**

- Calories: 85 kcal
- Fat: 11 g
- Carbohydrates: 2 g
- Proteins: 4 g

**Ingredients:**

- 1 green onion, chopped
- 1 large sweet potato, peeled
- 1 tsp. minced garlic

- 1-cup cilantro leaves
- 2-cup cauliflower florets
- ¼-tsp. ground black pepper
- ¼ tsp. salt
- ¼ cup sunflower seeds
- ¼ tsp. cumin
- ¼ cup ground flaxseed
- ½ tsp. red chili powder
- 2 tbsp. ranch seasoning mix
- 2 tbsp. arrowroot starch

## Directions:

1. Cut peeled sweet potato into small pieces, and then place them in a food processor and pulse until pieces are broken up.
2. Then add onion, cauliflower florets, and garlic, pulse until combined, add remaining ingredients and pulse more until incorporated.
3. Tip the mixture in a bowl, shape the mixture into seven 1 ½ inch thick patties, each about ¼ cup, then place them on a baking sheet and freeze for 10 minutes.
4. Switch on the air fryer, insert fryer basket, grease it with olive oil, then shut with its lid, set the fryer at 400°F and preheat for 10 minutes.

5.   Open the fryer, add patties in a single layer, close with its lid and cook for 20 minutes until nicely golden and cooked, flipping the patties halfway through the frying.

6.   When the air fryer beeps, open its lid, transfer patties onto a serving plate, and keep them warm.

7.   Cook the remaining patties in the same manner and serve.

# HASSEL BACK POTATOES

**Preparation Time:** 6 minutes

**Cooking Time:** 41 minutes

**Servings:** 2

## Nutritional values:

- Calories: 415
- Fat: 42 g
- Carbohydrates: 9 g
- Proteins: 1 g

## Ingredients:

1. 4 medium reddish potatoes washed and drained
2. 30 ml olive oil
3. 12 g salt
4. 1 g black pepper
5. 1 g garlic powder
6. 28 g melted butter
7. 8 g parsley, freshly chopped, to decorate

## Directions:

1. Wash and scrub potatoes. Let them dry with a paper towel.

2. Cut the slits, 6 mm away, on the potatoes, stopping before you cut them completely so that all the slices are connected approximately 13 mm at the bottom of the potato.

3. Preheat the air fryer for 6 minutes, set it to 175°C.

4. Cover the potatoes with olive oil and season evenly with salt, black pepper, and garlic powder.

5. Add the potatoes in the air fryer and cook for 30 minutes at 175°C.

6. Brush the melted butter over the potatoes and cook for another 10 minutes at 175°C.

7. Garnish with freshly chopped parsley.

# FRIED AVOCADO

**Preparation Time:** 9 minutes

**Cooking Time:** 10-15 minutes

**Servings:** 2

## Nutritional values:

- Calories: 123 kcal
- Fat: 11 g
- Carbohydrates: 2 g
- Proteins: 4 g

## Ingredients:

- 2 avocados cut into wedges 25 mm thick
- 50g Pan crumbs bread
- 2 g garlic powder
- 2 g onion powder
- 1 g smoked paprika
- 1 g cayenne pepper
- Salt and pepper to taste
- 60g all-purpose flour

- 2 eggs, beaten
- Nonstick Spray Oil
- Tomato sauce or ranch sauce, to serve

## Directions:

1. Cut the avocados into 25 mm thick pieces.
2. Combine the crumbs, garlic powder, onion powder, smoked paprika, cayenne pepper, and salt in a bowl.
3. Separate each wedge of avocado in the flour, then dip the beaten eggs and stir in the breadcrumb mixture.
4. Preheat the air fryer.
5. Place the avocados in the preheated air fryer baskets, spray with oil spray and cook at 205°C for 10 minutes. Turn the fried avocado halfway through cooking and sprinkle with cooking oil.

# *ONION FLOWER*

**Preparation Time:** 7 minutes

**Cooking Time:** 26 minutes

**Servings:** 3

## Nutritional values:

- Calories: 120 kcal
- Fat: 8.01 g
- Carbohydrates: 20.33 g
- Proteins: 1.98 g

## Ingredients:

- 1 large onion
- 120g all-purpose flour
- 7 g paprika
- 12 g salt
- 7 g garlic powder
- 3 g chili powder
- 1 g black pepper
- 1 g dried oregano

- 295 ml water
- 56 g Italian breadcrumbs
- Nonstick Spray Oil

**Directions:**

1. Peel the onion and cut the top. Place it on a cutting board. Cut down from the center out on the cutting board. Repeat to create 8 evenly separated cuts around the onion. Make sure your cut goes through all the layers, but leave the onion connected in the center. Leave aside.
2. Cover the onion in cold water for at least 2 hours and then dry it. Put the flour, paprika, salt, garlic powder, chili powder, black pepper, oregano, and water until a mixture forms.
3. Preheat the air fryer for 5 minutes at 180°C.
4. Cover the onion with the mixture, spread it over the layers, and make sure they are all covered. Then, sprinkle the top and bottom of the onion with the crumbs. Spray the bottom of the air fryer with cooking oil spray and place the onion inside cut up. Spray the top of the onion generously with oil spray.
5. Cook the onion at 205°C for 10 minutes, then cook for another 15 minutes at 175°C.

# SWEET POTATO SALT AND PEPPER

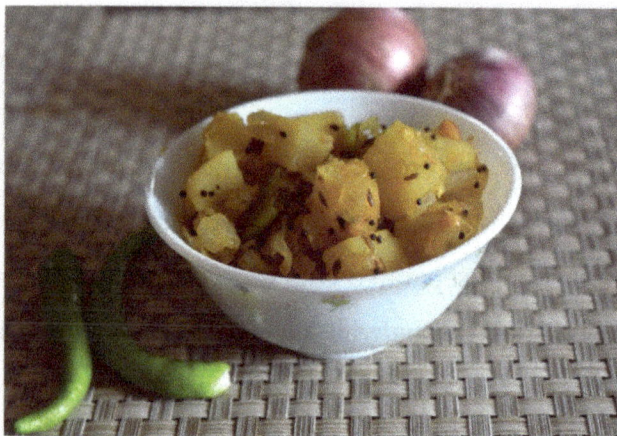

**Preparation Time:** 7 minutes

**Cooking Time:** 30-35 minutes

**Servings:** 4

## Nutritional values:

- Calories: 107 kcal
- Fat: 0.6 g
- Carbohydrates: 24.19 g
- Proteins: 1.61 g

## Ingredients:

- 1 large sweet potato
- Extra virgin olive oil
- Salt
- Ground pepper

## Directions:

1. Peel the sweet potato and cut it into thin strips; if you have a mandolin, it will be easier for you.

2. Wash well and put salt.

3. Add a little oil to impregnate the sweet potato in strips and place it in the air fryer basket.

4. Select 180°C, 30 minutes or so. From time to time, shake the basket so that the sweet potato moves.

5. Pass to a tray or plate and sprinkle with fine salt and ground pepper.

# *GARLICKY GREEN BEANS*

**Preparation Time:** 6 minutes

**Cooking Time:** 10-15 minutes

**Servings:** 4

**Nutritional values:**

- Calories: 45
- Fat: 11 g
- Carbohydrates: 2 g
- Proteins: 4 g

**Ingredients:**

- 1-pound green beans
- ¾-tsp. garlic powder
- ¾-tsp. ground black pepper
- 1 ¼-tsp. salt
- ½-tsp. paprika

## Directions:

1. Switch on the air fryer, insert fryer basket, grease it with olive oil, then shut with its lid, set the fryer at 400°F and preheat for 5 minutes.

2. Meanwhile, place beans in a bowl, spray generously with olive oil, sprinkle with garlic powder, black pepper, salt, and paprika and toss until well coated.

3. Open the fryer, add green beans in it, close with its lid and cook for 8 minutes until nicely golden and crispy, shaking halfway through the frying.

4. When the air fryer beeps, open its lid, transfer green beans onto a serving plate and serve.

# CRISPY RYE BREAD SNACKS WITH GUACAMOLE AND ANCHOVIES

**Preparation Time:** 12 minutes

**Cooking Time:** 8 minutes

**Servings:** 4

## Nutritional values:

- Calories: 180 kcal
- Fat: 11 g
- Carbohydrates: 4 g
- Proteins: 4 g

## Ingredients:

- 4 slices rye bread
- Guacamole
- Anchovies in oil

## Directions:

1. Cut each slice of bread into 3 strips of bread.
2. Place in the air fryer's basket without piling up, and we go in batches giving it the touch you want to give it. You can select 180°C, 10 minutes.
3. When you have all the crusty rye bread strips, put a layer of guacamole on top, whether homemade or commercial.
4. In each bread, place 2 anchovies on the guacamole.

# *VEGETABLES IN AIR FRYER*

**Preparation Time:** 6 minutes

**Cooking Time:** 31 minutes

**Servings:** 2

## Nutritional values:

- Calories: 135 kcal
- Fat: 11 g
- Carbohydrates: 2 g
- Proteins: 4 g

## Ingredients:

- 2 potatoes
- 1 zucchini
- 1 onion
- 1 red pepper
- 1 green pepper

## Directions:

1. Cut the potatoes into slices.
2. Cut the onion into rings.
3. Cut the zucchini slices
4. Cut the peppers into strips.
5. Put all the ingredients in the bowl and add a little salt, ground pepper, and some extra virgin olive oil.
6. Mix well.
7. Pass to the basket of the air fryer.
8. Select 160°C, 30 minutes.
9. Check that the vegetables are to your liking.

# *AIR FRYER SUGAR-FREE LEMON SLICE AND BAKE COOKIES*

**Preparation Time:** 5 minutes

**Cooking Time:** 8 minutes

**Servings:** 24

## Nutritional values:

- Calories: 66 kcal
- Fat: 6 g
- Carbohydrates: 2 g
- Proteins: 1 g

## Ingredients:

- ½ tsp. salt
- ½ cup coconut flour
- ½ cup unsalted butter softened

- ½ tsp. liquid vanilla stevia
- ½ cup swerve granular sweetener
- 1 tbsp. lemon juice
- ¼ tsp. lemon extract (optional)
- 2 egg yolks

For icing

- 3 tsp. lemon juice
- 2/3 cup Swerve confectioner's sweetener

## Directions:

1. In a stand mixer bowl, add baking soda, coconut flour, salt, and Swerve, mix until well combined

2. Then add the butter (softened) to the dry ingredient, mix well. Add all the remaining ingredients but do not add in the yolks yet. Adjust the seasoning of lemon flavor and sweetness to your liking; add more if needed.

3. Add the yolk and combine well.

4. Lay a big piece of plastic wrap on a flat surface, put the batter in the center, roll around the dough and make it into a log form for almost 12 inches. Keep this log in the fridge for 2–3 hours or overnight, if possible.

5. Let the oven preheat to 325°F. generously spray the air fryer basket, take the log out from plastic wrap, only

unwrap how much you want to use it, and keep the rest in the fridge.

6. Cut in ¼-inch cookies, place as many cookies in the air fryer basket in one single, do not overcrowd the basket.

7. Bake for 3-five minutes, or until the cookies' edges become brown. Let it cool in the basket for two minutes, then take it out from the basket. And let them cool on a wire rack.

8. Once all cookies are baked, pour the icing over. Serve and enjoy.

# EASY AIR FRYER BROWNIES

**Preparation Time:** 9 minutes

**Cooking Time:** 10 minutes

**Servings:** 2

**Nutritional values:**

- Calories: 201 kcal
- Fat: 10.2 g
- Carbohydrates: 14.1 g
- Proteins: 8.7 g

**Ingredients:**

- 2 tbsp. baking chips
- 1/3 cup almond flour
- 1 egg
- ½ tsp. baking powder
- 3 tbsp. powdered sweetener (sugar alternative)
- 2 tbsp. cocoa powder (Unsweetened)
- 2 tbsp. chopped Pecans
- 4 tbsp. melted butter

## Directions:

1. Let the air fryer preheat to 350°F

2. In a large bowl, add cocoa powder, almond flour, Swerve sugar substitute, and baking powder, and give it a good mix.

3. Add melted butter and crack in the egg in the dry ingredients.

4. Mix well until combined and smooth.

5. Fold in the chopped pecans and baking chips.

6. Take two ramekins to grease them well with softened butter. Add the batter to them.

7. Bake for ten minutes. Make sure to place them as far from the heat source from the top in the air fryer.

8. Take the brownies out from the air fryer and let them cool for five minutes.

9. Serve with your favorite toppings and enjoy.

# *AIR FRYER THUMBPRINT COOKIES*

**Preparation Time:** 15 minutes

**Cooking Time:** 8 minutes

**Servings:** 10

**Nutritional values:**

- Calories: 111.6
- Fat: 8.6 g
- Carbohydrates: 9.1 g
- Proteins: 3.7 g

**Ingredients:**

- 1 tsp. baking powder
- 1 cup almond flour
- 3 tbsp. natural low-calorie sweetener
- 1 large egg
- 3 and a half tbsp. raspberry (reduced-sugar) preserves
- 4 tbsp. softened cream cheese

## Directions:

1.  In a large bowl, add egg, baking powder, flour, sweetener, and cream cheese, mix well until a dough (wet) forms.
2.  Chill the dough in the fridge for almost 20 minutes, until dough is cool enough
3.  And then form into balls.
4.  Let the air fryer preheat to 400°F, add the parchment paper to the air fryer basket.
5.  Make ten balls from the dough and put them in the prepared air fryer basket.
6.  With your clean hands, make an indentation from your thumb in the center of every cookie. Add one tsp. of the raspberry preserve in the thumb hole.
7.  Bake in the air fryer for seven minutes or until light golden brown to your liking.
8.  Let the cookies cool completely in the parchment paper for almost 15 minutes, or they will fall apart.
9.  Serve with tea and enjoy.

# *AIR FRYER APPLE FRITTER*

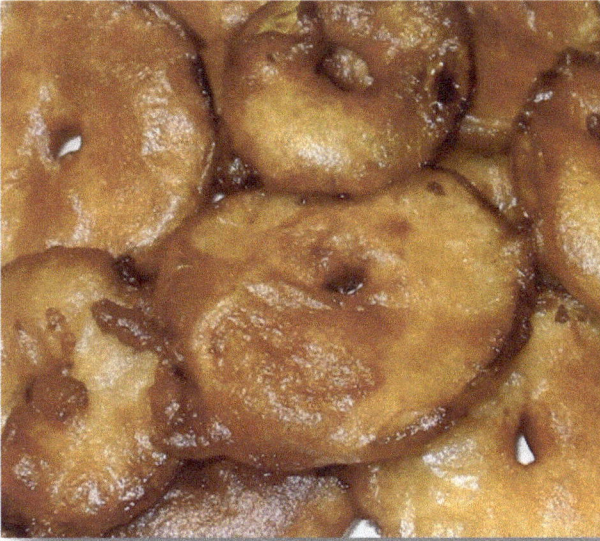

**Preparation Time:** 9 minutes

**Cooking Time:** 15 minutes

**Servings:** 3

## Nutritional values:

- Calories: 200 kcal
- Fat: 12 g
- Carbohydrates: 14 g
- Proteins: 9.8 g

## Ingredients:

- ½ apple (Pink Lady Apple or Honey crisp) peeled, finely chopped
- ½ cup all-purpose flour
- 1 tsp. baking powder
- ¼ tsp. Kosher salt
- ½ tsp. ground cinnamon
- 2 tbsp. brown sugar or sugar alternative
- 1/8 tsp. ground nutmeg
- 3 tbsp. Greek yogurt (Fat -Free)
- 1 tbsp. butter

For the glaze:

- 2 tbsp. powdered sugar
- ½ tbsp. water

## Directions:

1. In a big mixing bowl, add baking powder, nutmeg, brown sugar (or alternative), flour, cinnamon, and salt. Mix it well,

2. With the help of a fork or cutter, slice the butter until crumbly. It should look like wet sand.

3. Add the chopped apple and coat well, then add fat-free Greek yogurt.

4.  Keep stirring or tossing until everything together, and a crumbly dough forms.

5.  Put the dough on a clean surface and with your hands, knead it into a ball form.

6.  Flatten the dough in an oval shape about a half-inch thick. It is okay, even if it's not the perfect size or shape.

7.  Spray the basket of the air fryer with cooking spray generously. Put the dough in the air fry for 12–14 minutes at 375°F cook until light golden brown.

8.  For making the glaze mix, the ingredients, and with the help of a brush, pour over the apple fritter when it comes out from the air fryer.

9.  Slice and serve after cooling for 5 minutes.

# *BERRY CHEESECAKE*

**Preparation Time:** 9 minutes

**Cooking Time:** 51 minutes

**Servings:** 8

## Nutritional values:

- Calories: 225 kcal
- Fat: 17 g
- Carbohydrates: 18 g
- Proteins: 12 g

## Ingredients:

- ½cup raspberries
- 2 blocks of softened cream cheese, 8 ounces
- 1 tsp. raspberry or vanilla extract
- ¼ cup strawberries
- 2 eggs
- ¼ cup blackberries
- One cup and 2 tbsp. sugar alternative of confectioner sweetener

## Directions:

1.  In a big mixing bowl, whip the sugar-alternative confectioner sweetener and cream cheese, mix whip until smooth and creamy.

2.  Then add in the raspberry or vanilla extract and eggs, again mix well.

3.  In a food processor or a blender, pulse the berries and fold into the cream cheese mix with two extra tbsp. of sweetener.

4.  Take a springform pan and spray the oil generously, pour in the mixture.

5.  Put the pan in the air fryer, let it air fryer, and cook for ten minutes at 300°F. Lower the temperature to 400°F and cook for 40 minutes.

6.  To check if it's done, shake it lightly. If everything is set and the middle part is jiggled, it is done.

7.  Take out from the air fryer and cool a bit before chilling in the fridge.

8.  Keep in the fridge for 2–4 hours or as long as you have time.

9.  Slice and serve, enjoy.

# *GRAIN-FREE MOLTEN LAVA CAKES*

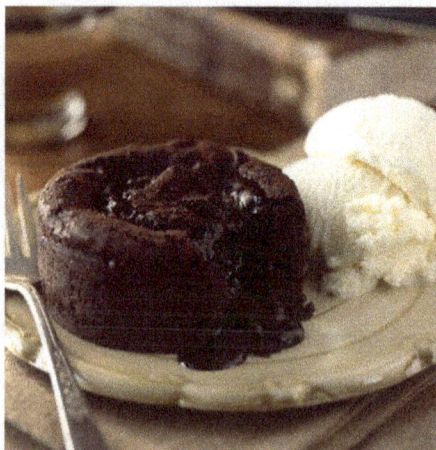

**Preparation Time:** 5 minutes

**Cooking Time:** 10-15 minutes

**Servings:** 2

**Nutritional values:**

- Calories: 217 kcal
- Fat: 12 g
- Carbohydrates: 14 g
- Proteins: 9.9 g

## Ingredients:

- 2 large eggs
- 1/2 cup chocolate chips, you can use dark chocolate
- 2 tbsp. coconut flour
- 2 tbsp. honey as a sugar substitute
- A dash sea salt
- ½ tsp. baking soda
- Butter and cocoa powder (for two small ramekins)
- ¼ cup butter or grass-fed butter

## Directions:

1. Let the air fryer preheat to 370°F.
2. Grease the ramekins with soft butter and sprinkle with cocoa powder. It will stick to the butter. Turn the ramekins upside down, so excess cocoa powder will fall out. Set it aside.
3. In a double boiler or microwave, safe bowl, melt the butter and chocolate chips together, stir every 15 seconds. Make sure to mix well to combine.
4. In a large bowl, crack the eggs and whisk with either honey or sugar, mix well. Add in the baking soda, sea salt, and coconut flour. Gently fold everything.

5. Then add the melted chocolate chip and butter mixture to the egg, flour, and honey mixture. Mix well, so everything combines.

6. Pour the batter in those two prepared ramekins.

7. Let them air fry for ten minutes. Then take them out from the air fryer and let them cool for 3 to 4 minutes.

8. When cool enough to handle, run a knife along the edges so the cake will out easier.

9. After flipping them upside down on a serving plate.

10. Top with mint leaves and coconut cream, raspberries, if you want. Serve right away and enjoy.